TAIGAN DOG

The Ultimate Handbook To Raising A Well-Behaved Taigan Dog For Beginners

CARL JUAN

Table of Contents

Introductory

Originally from Kyrgyzstan, the Taigan dog breed is prized for its keen eyesight. This dog's genetic make-up lends itself to hunting by sight and speed, making it a sighthound. The Taigan people are well-known for their prowess in tracking and capturing game animals. They are typically used to hunt hares, foxes, and other small to medium-sized animals in the mountainous regions of Kyrgyzstan due to their slim, athletic form.

The Taigan dog is linked to the Kazakh Tazi, another type of sighthound. The Kyrgyz people hold these dogs in the highest regard for both their hunting skills and their companionship. They stand out from the crowd thanks to their sleek coat and refined demeanor.

Taigan dogs are well-known not just for their prowess as hunters, but also for the dedication and devotion they show their human companions. If you understand and respect their individuality and are able to give them the exercise and attention they require, they can be wonderful companions.

CHAPTER ONE
Taigan Selection

Choosing a dog, be it a Taigan or another breed, is a huge responsibility. Here are some things to keep in mind while you search for a Taigan:

• First, you should do as much research as possible on the Taigan breed. Think about what they're like, what they need, and how they act. Verify if the characteristics of the breed you're considering are consistent with your own ideals.

• Trustworthy Breeder: Try to locate a reliable breeder who focuses on Taigan canines. The health and happiness of their dogs comes first for a conscientious breeder, and they know what each breed needs to thrive.

• Inquire about the health clearances and screening results of the puppy's parents from the breeder. This can involve assessments for prevalent breed-specific health concerns. For the sake of the puppy's future health, it's crucial to find a breeder who does genetic testing.

• Get to Know the Parents: If at all feasible, meet the puppy's mom and dad. This can shed light on the canine ancestry's typical personality traits.

• Don't be shy about questioning the breeder about the puppies' care, breeding techniques, and anything else you can think of. A trustworthy breeder will not hide any information regarding their breeding practices.

• If at all possible, it's a good idea to visit a breeder and watch firsthand how the puppies are cared for and how they interact with their surroundings. You may gauge the breeder's dedication to the dogs' well-being based on this.

• Make sure the puppies have been well socialized from the time they are very young. Taigan puppies need early and consistent socialization to mature into happy, healthy dogs.

• Puppies from ethical breeders come with a health guarantee that protects buyers against the costs of specific medical conditions for a set length of time. Make sure you understand the terms of the warranty.

• Think About Your Daily Routine, Activity Level, and Where You Live. Because of their high energy levels,

Taigans require daily walks and playtime to stay happy and healthy.

• The time and energy you put into training and caring for your Taigan is well worth it. These canines are very trainable given the right direction and socialization.

• Think about whether you'd rather get a Taigan from a rescue group or a breeder-raised puppy. There are benefits and drawbacks to both choices.

Getting a dog is a long-term commitment, so keep in mind that the Taigan breed has specific needs. Ensure you're ready for this commitment before introducing a Taigan into your life.

Material Requirements

There are a few things you absolutely must have on hand when you adopt a Taigan, or any dog, into your home. The following items are required for your Taigan:

1. Bowls for Food and Drinking Water Stainless steel or ceramic bowls are long-lasting and simple to clean.

2. Premium Dog Food: Feed your Taigan a premium dog food that is formulated for his or her age, size, and level of activity. If you need advice, talk to your vet.

3. Walks and identification both require a collar and ID tag, as well as a strong leash.

4. Give your Taigan a soft place to sleep, like a bed or a kennel.

5. Crate or Kennel: A crate can serve as a safe and secure area for your dog, especially during training and transport.

6. Toys: Stock up on entertaining and thought-provoking options.

7. Brushes, combs, and other grooming items may be necessary, depending on the coat type of your Taigan. Maintaining the health of their coat relies on regular care.

8. Dog-specific shampoo, towels, and a tub or other space set aside for bathing should be on hand.

9. If you want to know how to protect your pet against fleas and ticks, consult your veterinarian.

10. Get on a heartworm prevention program after discussing it with your vet.

11. Bags to collect dog waste on walks and other outdoor excursions are called "doggy poop bags."

12. If you intend to train your Taigan, you will need training treats, a clicker, and other training equipment.

13. You should get a dog license and make sure your dog wears identifying tags with your contact information.

14. A standard first aid pack for use on pets in the event of accidents or medical problems.

15. Care for your dog's teeth with a dog-sized toothbrush and canine-formulated toothpaste.

16. Food & Treat Storage: Containers help keep your dog's food fresh and accessible.

17. Pack a travel crate, harness, or seatbelt restraint for your dog if you're going on a trip with him.

18. Keep your Taigan safe by familiarizing yourself with this list of hazardous plants and common household hazards.

19. Books on training and behavior might help you better understand and manage your dog.

20. Establish a working connection with a trusted local vet and take advantage of routine checkups and immunizations.

It's vital to note that your dog's demands may alter as they grow and age, so frequently review and update your supplies to fit their changing requirements. Make sure your Taigan gets lots of affection, playtime, and exercise to keep it content and healthy.

CHAPTER TWO
Nutrition and Health in Taigan

Keeping your Taigan in good shape through proper diet and exercise is crucial if you want them to live a long and fulfilling life. For the sake of Taigan health and nutrition, please follow these rules:

1. Top-Notch Dog Treats:

• Feed your Taigan a high-quality kibble that's suitable for his or her age, size, and level of activity. Find formulas that use premium protein sources.

2. Scheduled Mealtimes:

• Spread your dog's daily rations out over the course of two or three meals. Adult dogs only need to eat twice daily, but puppies need to eat three or four times a day.

3. Food Portions:

• Give your Taigan the same amount of food every day as indicated on the dog food bag, but always take into account your pet's unique dietary requirements. Modify serving quantities according to your dog's age, size, and activity level.

4. True Hydration:

• Maintain a constant supply of potable water for your Taigan.

5. Never Accept Free Food:

• Free-feeding, or leaving food out all day, can cause people to overeat and gain weight. Try to eat at regular intervals.

6. Diet High in Protein:

• Taigans do best on a diet high in animal products including meat, fish, and fowl. They rely on protein to maintain lean muscle mass and an active lifestyle.

7. Nutritional Fats:

• For healthy skin and a shiny coat, incorporate good fats into their diet, like those found in fish or flaxseed oil.

8. Cut out the Fluff:

• Feed your dog a diet low in fillers like corn, wheat, and soy. The nutritional value of these ingredients is low.

9. Track Mass:

• Be aware of how much your Taigan weighs. Health problems arise for overweight dogs. You may need to make some changes to their diet and exercise routine.

10. Taigans are energetic dogs that require regular playtime to stay healthy. Exercising and playing daily is crucial.

11. Animal Health: Have your vet examine your pet regularly. Maintain a regular schedule of immunizations, flea/tick treatment, and heartworm medication.

12. Care for your Taigan's teeth by giving it dental chews or toys and giving it a regular brushing.

13. Special Dietary Considerations: - If your Taigan has special dietary requirements or food allergies, you should seek advice from your veterinarian before making any food choices.

14. Chocolate, grapes, and some artificial sweeteners, such as xylitol, are toxic to dogs and should be avoided at all costs.

15. Weight Management: - If your Taigan becomes overweight, work with your vet to develop a weight management plan, which may include dietary adjustments and increased exercise.

Depending on your Taigan's age, level of activity, and general health, they may have different dietary needs. To give your dog the best care possible, it's a good idea to work with your vet to develop a unique diet and health regimen just for them.

Workouts and Conditioning

Care for a Taigan must include regular training and exercise. These smart and energetic canines need plenty of exercise and mental challenge to stay happy and healthy. The following are suggestions for training and exercising your Taigan:

Exercise:

• Because of their high energy levels, Taigans require daily walks or runs. Exercise for at least an hour, preferably two. Walking, running, and other forms of physical activity are acceptable here.

• **Play without a Leash:** Offer off-leash playtime in a safe, fenced area. Taigans get to exercise their sighthound instincts by engaging in their favorite pastime, which is running and chasing.

• Taigans can also benefit from mental stimulation in addition to physical exercise. Obedience training, puzzle feeders, and interactive toys can all help to keep pets mentally stimulated.

• Provide a wide range of entertainment options to ward off boredom. This can include hiking, agility training, and even dog sports like lure coursing.

• It's important to start socializing young and keep it up throughout life. Make sure your Taigan is well-adjusted and at ease in a variety of settings by exposing it to a wide range of people, animals, and environments.

Training:

• Rewards for good behavior in training should take the form of positive reinforcement, such as treats, praise, and toys. Do not use punishment as a form of discipline.

• **Obedience Training:** Taigans should be taught the basics of obedience, including how to sit, stay, come, and heel. This is for both their own security and your own peace of mind.

• **Consistency:** Maintain a regular training schedule. Always reward good behavior and issue clear commands.

- As was previously mentioned, Taigans rely heavily on their social interactions. To avoid problems with fear or aggression later on, socialize them early and often with a variety of people, animals, and environments.

- Training on a leash is recommended for Taigans because of their high prey drive; otherwise, they might run after small animals on walks.

- Training your Taigan to come when called off-leash requires a solid recall command. This is a must if they are to avoid harm.

• If you're having trouble training your Taigan, you might want to look into dog training classes or hiring a professional dog trainer.

• Training may take some time, so try to keep a positive outlook and persevere through the process. Dogs learn best in an upbeat, positive environment.

Keep in mind that training can be more difficult with a Taigan because of their intelligence and independence. A well-behaved and content Taigan is possible with the right amount of time, effort, and praise.

CHAPTER THREE
Taigan Maintenance

The health and happiness of your Taigan depends on regular grooming. The specific coat type and the dog's lifestyle will determine how often the dog needs to be groomed, but in general, Taigans have a dense double coat that requires regular maintenance. A few notes on Taigan grooming:

1. Brushing:

The Taigan's double coat is thick and warm. Maintaining a healthy coat requires regular brushing to remove dead hair, prevent mats, and disperse the coat's natural oils.

Your Taigan needs to be brushed several times weekly, and more frequently during shedding seasons.

2. Bathing:

• Unless they get very dirty, Taigans don't need to be washed very often. Avoid skin problems by using a dog-specific shampoo and carefully rinsing and drying the coat afterward.

3. De-Matting and Detangling:

• Pay special attention to the back of the neck and the area behind the ears, as these are common places for mats to form. Use a slicker brush or mat splitter to gently remove the knots from these spots.

4. Ears:

Avoid ear infections by keeping a close eye on and cleaning their ears frequently. Use a cotton swab and ear cleaning solution recommended by your vet; just be careful not to force anything deeper into the ear canal.

5. Nails:

Nails should be trimmed when they get too long to avoid pain and injury. Have a professional groomer or veterinarian show you how to do it if you're unsure.

6. Oral Health:

Maintain your Taigan's healthy smile by giving it regular tooth brushings. Dog-friendly alternatives to human toothpaste and toothbrushes can be found for this purpose.

7. Insuring Proper Vision:

You should clean their eyes whenever there is discharge or dust. To clean your dog's eyes, use a damp, clean cloth or doggie wipes.

8. Preserving Your Coat:

• Take note of the coat's overall health. Check the skin for fleas, ticks, or other skin problems. If you notice any problems, consult with your veterinarian.

9. Shedding:

• Taigans, like many other animals, shed their skin periodically. You should use a deshedding tool or brush to deal with the extra fur that will fall out during these times.

10. Expert Barbering:

• If you're not sure you can give your Taigan a good grooming on your own, it might be worth it to take it to a professional groomer, especially if they need their coat trimmed.

11. Keep the Area Tidy and Clean:

To control the hair that is falling out, you should regularly clean and vacuum. To preserve the condition of your furniture, use a furniture cover or a rug.

It's best to begin training your Taigan at a young age so they can adjust to the routine. It's a good idea to look for signs of skin problems and other health problems during your regular grooming sessions. Your Taigan will appreciate it if you attend to their coat and other grooming needs on a regular basis.

In the right home, a Taigan can become a wonderful member of the family. If you want your relationship with them to be successful and harmonious, you need to learn about their individual needs and quirks. **If you're thinking about adopting a Taigan, here are some things to think about:**

1. Active Lifestyle: Taigans are active dogs with a strong prey drive. They enjoy running and playing, and they require regular exercise to stay healthy and happy. If your family leads an active lifestyle and can provide ample exercise and playtime for your Taigan, they can be a good fit.

2. **Socialization:** Proper socialization is essential from a young age. Taigans should be exposed to various people, animals, and environments to ensure they are well-adjusted and comfortable in different situations. Early socialization helps them get along well with children and other pets.

3. Supervision with Children: Taigans can be good with children when properly socialized and raised with them. However, like any dog, they should be supervised when interacting with young children to prevent accidental injuries, as they can be quite energetic and have a strong prey drive.

4. Grooming Commitment: Be prepared for regular grooming and shedding. Taigans have a dense double coat that requires regular brushing to prevent matting and minimize shedding.

5. Training and Obedience: Taigans are intelligent but independent dogs. Consistent and positive reinforcement-based training is essential to ensure they are well-behaved family members. They may be a bit more challenging to train than some other breeds, but with patience and consistent training, they can be obedient and well-mannered.

6. Space: While Taigans can adapt to apartment living with sufficient exercise, they often do better in homes with access to a yard where they can run and play.

7. Prey Drive: Keep in mind that Taigans have a strong prey drive, which means they may chase small animals. It's essential to train them to have a reliable recall and use a leash when walking them in areas with wildlife.

8. Professional Help: If you're new to dog ownership or have specific concerns, consider working with a professional dog trainer or behaviorist to ensure a smooth transition of your Taigan into a family environment.

9. Time and Commitment: Owning any dog, including Taigans, requires time, attention, and care. Be prepared for a long-term commitment to their well-being.

In summary, Taigans can be great family pets when they are provided with the right environment, training, and socialization. If you have an active family, can meet their exercise needs, and are willing to invest time in grooming and training, a Taigan can be a loyal and loving addition to your family. However, always consider the individual temperament and needs of the dog, and ensure that they are a good fit for your family's lifestyle and expectations.

CHAPTER FOUR
Activities and Enrichment

Keeping your Taigan mentally and physically stimulated is essential to prevent boredom and ensure their well-being. Taigans are active dogs with strong instincts, so providing them with a variety of activities and enrichment can help channel their energy in a positive way. Here are some activities and enrichment ideas for your Taigan:

• **Outdoor Adventures:** Taigans love to run and explore. Take them on hikes, long walks, or trips to a dog-friendly beach or park. These outings allow them to use their natural instincts and get the exercise they need.

• **Play Fetch:** Taigans often enjoy a good game of fetch. Use a ball or toy to play fetch with them in a safely enclosed area.

• **Interactive Toys:** Provide interactive toys that dispense treats when your Taigan figures out how to get them. This stimulates their problem-solving skills and keeps them mentally engaged.

• **Puzzle Feeders:** Use puzzle feeders to make mealtime more interesting. These devices challenge your dog to work for their food, providing mental stimulation.

• **Obedience Training:** Taigans are intelligent and can excel in obedience training. Enroll them in training classes or engage in regular training sessions to reinforce good behavior and teach new commands.

• **Nose Work:** Taigans have a keen sense of smell. Engage their noses by hiding treats or toys around the house or yard for them to find.

• **Agility Training:** Set up a mini agility course in your backyard or attend agility classes. Taigans can excel in agility, and it provides both mental and physical exercise.

• **Lure Coursing:** Consider trying lure coursing, a sport that simulates chasing prey. Taigans excel at this activity and love the opportunity to run.

• **Playdates:** Arrange playdates with other well-behaved dogs for social interaction and exercise.

• **Tug of War:** Taigans can enjoy a game of tug of war with a sturdy rope toy. Ensure that the game is played safely and with clear rules.

• **Dog Sports:** Consider getting involved in dog sports such as flyball, Canine Freestyle, or dock diving, depending on your Taigan's interests and abilities.

• **Mental Challenges:** Create mental challenges by teaching your Taigan new tricks, providing them with puzzle toys, and varying their daily routines to keep their minds engaged.

• **Hide and Seek:** Play hide and seek with your Taigan. Hide and call them to find you. This game engages their tracking skills and is fun for both of you.

• **Relaxation Time:** Taigans need downtime too. Make sure they have a comfortable place to rest and relax after their activities.

- **Doggy Daycare:** If you're away during the day, consider doggy daycare as a way to keep your Taigan mentally and physically active in a supervised environment.

Remember that mental and physical exercise is crucial for Taigans to prevent behavioral issues and ensure their well-being. Tailor their activities to their specific interests and energy level, and always supervise them during playtime to ensure their safety.

Breeding Considerations

Breeding a dog is a significant responsibility and should only be undertaken with careful consideration, ethical intentions, and a deep understanding of the breed's specific needs and traits. If you are considering breeding Taigans, here are some important factors and considerations to keep in mind:

1. Breed Standard: Ensure your Taigans conform to the breed standard in terms of appearance, temperament, and health. Dogs used for breeding should be of exceptional quality and free from any hereditary health issues.

2. Health Screening: Conduct comprehensive health screenings on potential breeding dogs, including genetic tests for common breed-specific conditions. This helps reduce the risk of passing on hereditary diseases to offspring.

3. Pedigree and Lineage: Study the pedigrees of the dogs you plan to breed to understand their lineage and genetics. A good breeder strives to improve the breed with each generation and maintains detailed records of their dogs' lineage.

4. Temperament: Select breeding dogs with stable and desirable temperaments. Dogs with aggressive or anxious tendencies should not be used for breeding.

5. Age and Health: Ensure that both the male and female dogs are in prime health and condition. Breeding dogs should be at an appropriate age, and females should not be bred on their first or last heat cycle.

6. Ethical Breeding Practices: Always prioritize the welfare of the dogs involved. Avoid excessive breeding, and give breeding dogs appropriate rest between litters.

Overbreeding can be harmful to the health of the female dog.

7. Whelping and Puppy Care: Be prepared to provide proper care for the pregnant female and newborn puppies, including appropriate veterinary care, socialization, and nutrition.

8. Placement of Puppies: Be committed to finding responsible and loving homes for the puppies. Screen potential puppy buyers to ensure they are capable of providing a good home.

9. Legal Requirements: Familiarize yourself with local and national breeding regulations and ensure you comply with all necessary permits and laws.

10. Breeding Mentorship: It's beneficial to seek guidance and mentorship from experienced breeders. They can provide valuable advice and support as you start your breeding program.

11. Responsible Advertising: If you decide to breed, ensure any advertising is honest and accurate, and avoid sensationalism. Ethical breeders prioritize the well-being of the dogs and the breed itself.

12. Continued Education: Stay up-to-date with advancements in breeding, health, and genetics. Attend seminars and conferences to continually improve your breeding program.

Breeding dogs is a significant commitment, and it should not be entered into lightly. It's important to have a genuine passion for the breed, a commitment to their well-being, and a dedication to improving the breed's overall health and temperament. Always put the dogs' welfare above any financial gain, and be prepared for the responsibilities of breeding, including the possibility of needing to care for puppies throughout their lives if they cannot find suitable homes. Additionally, consider whether there are already enough Taigans in need of homes in your area and whether breeding is truly necessary.

Taigan in Different Environments

Taigans, being a versatile breed with strong sighthound traits, can adapt to different environments, but their specific needs and challenges can vary depending on the environment. Here's how Taigans can thrive in various settings:

1. Urban Environment:

• **Exercise:** Taigans can adapt to urban living but require daily exercise. Regular walks, trips to the dog park, and playtime in designated areas are essential.

• **Space:** Access to a small yard or a nearby park can provide opportunities for exercise.

• **Socialization:** Early and ongoing socialization is crucial in urban areas, as your Taigan will encounter various people, dogs, and stimuli.

2. Suburban or Residential Area:

• **Yard:** Having a yard is ideal for Taigans to run and play. Ensure it is securely gated, as Taigans have a high predatory drive.

• **Workout:** Take advantage of neighboring parks and trails for more workout opportunities.

• **Socialization:** Suburban locations typically have other dogs, which can be beneficial for socialization.

3. Rural Environment:

• **Space:** Rural areas can be great for Taigans due to the wide space. However, still, have a sturdy fence as they may be more tempted to hunt wildlife.

- **Exercise:** Taigans can thrive in rural regions with plenty of open grounds for running.

- **Hunting:** In some rural locations, Taigans may be employed for hunting small game.

4. Country or Farm Setting:

- **Working Dogs:** Taigans are occasionally used as working dogs on farms and in rural locations to guard animals and hunt vermin.

• **Exercise:** They can appreciate the open spaces and the opportunity to employ their natural inclinations.

5. Mountainous Terrain:

• **Exercise:** Taigans can adapt to high terrain and may thrive in sports like trekking and climbing. Be mindful of their exercise limits at higher elevations.

6. Hot Climates:

• **Hydration:** In hot areas, be particularly careful to their hydration. Ensure they have access to fresh water and avoid intense exercise during the hottest times of the day.

• **Shade:** Provide shade and restrict sun exposure, as Taigans can be prone to overheating.

7. Cold Climates:

• **Cold Weather Gear:** In cold locations, consider utilizing protective clothes for your Taigan, such as a dog coat. Their short coat may require more insulation during chilly weather.

In all circumstances, it's crucial to pay attention to your Taigan's individual demands, such as grooming and exercise. Regular grooming, including brushing and coat maintenance, is necessary to protect them from environmental hazards. Socialization remains vital in every context to ensure they are well-adjusted and comfortable in diverse scenarios.

Remember that each Taigans may have their own preferences and adaptability. Observe and adjust to their requirements and personality to give the best possible living environment for your dog.

Conclusion

Taigans are a unique breed of sighthound that can make fantastic companions for the appropriate people. These dogs are recognized for their agility, speed, and hunting abilities, but they also have a devoted and friendly personality. If you're considering introducing a Taigan into your life, here are the essential takeaways:

1. Investigate & Preparation: Before getting a Taigan, extensively investigate the breed to verify it's a good fit for your lifestyle and interests. Be prepared for the responsibility of caring for this active and intellectual breed.

2. Health and Nutrition: Provide a high-quality diet, frequent exercise, and veterinarian treatment to keep your Taigan healthy. Grooming and frequent check-ups are also crucial.

3. Exercise and Training: Taigans need both physical and mental stimulation. Regular exercise and positive reinforcement-based training are vital for their well-being.

4. Family Pet: Taigans can be terrific family pets provided you have an active lifestyle, give proper socialization, and watch their interactions with children and other pets.

5. Breeding Considerations: Breeding should be undertaken with care, responsibility, and a commitment to the welfare of the dogs involved. Ethical breeding procedures are vital.

6. Activities and Enrichment: Keep your Taigan mentally and physically busy with diverse activities and enrichment to prevent boredom.

7. Adaptation to settings: Taigans can adjust to different settings, although their individual demands and problems may vary. Pay attention to their specific demands and adapt accordingly.

Remember that having a Taigan is a long-term commitment that demands devotion, patience, and love. With the correct care and attention, these loyal and clever dogs can be a great addition to your family and give you with years of company and joy.

THE END

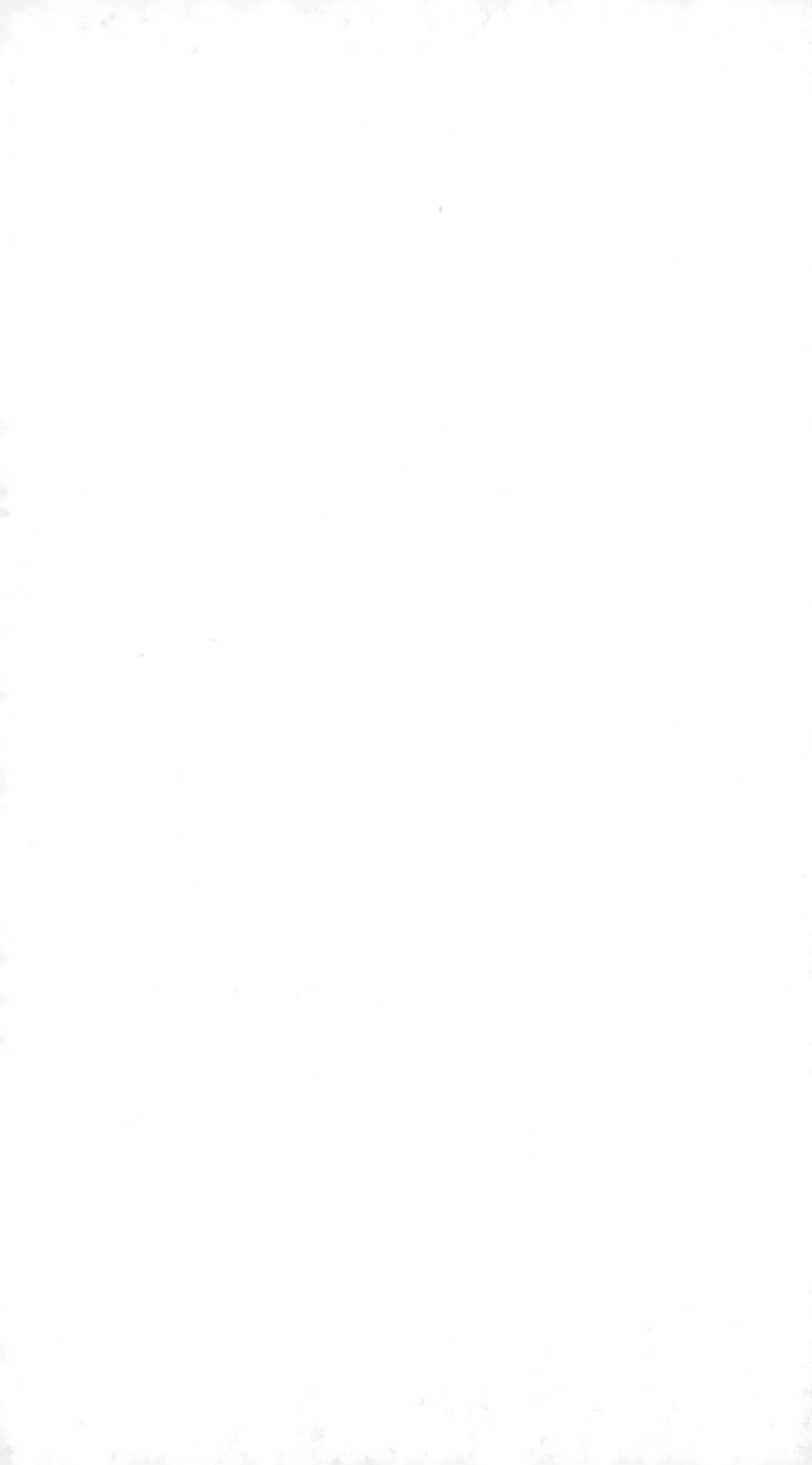